Preventive and Community Dentistry

Clinical Record Book

Preventive and Community Dentistry Clinical Record Book

M Shivakumar
MDS
Professor and Head
Department of Community Dentistry
Ragas Dental College and Hospital
Chennai

JAYPEE BROTHERS
MEDICAL PUBLISHERS (P) LTD
New Delhi

Published by
Jitendar P Vij
Jaypee Brothers Medical Publishers (P) Ltd
EMCA House, 23/23B Ansari Road, Daryaganj
New Delhi 110 002, India
Phones: +91-11-23272143, +91-11-23272703, +91-11-23282021, +91-11-23245672
Fax: +91-11-23276490, +91-11-23245683 e-mail: jaypee@jaypeebrothers.com
Visit our website: www.jaypeebrothers.com

Branches

- 2/B Akruti Society, Jodhpur Gam Road, Satellite, **Ahmedabad** 380 015
  Phone: +91-079-30988717, +91-079-26926233 e-mail: jpandvd@rediffmail.com
- 202 Batavia Chambers, 8 Kumara Krupa Road, Kumara Park East,
  Bangalore 560 001, Phones: +91-80-22285971, +91-80-22382956, +91-80-30614073
  Tele Fax: +91-80-22281761 e-mail: jaypeemedpubbgl@eth.net
- 282 IIIrd Floor, Khaleel Shirazi Estate, Fountain Plaza, Pantheon Road
  Chennai 600 008, Phones: +91-44-28262665, +91-44-28269897, +91-44-030972089
  Fax: +91-44-28262331 e-mail: jpchen@eth.net
- 4-2-1067/1-3, Ist Floor, Balaji Building, Ramkote, Cross Road
  Hyderabad 500 095, Phones: +91-40-55610020, +91-40-24758498, +91-40-30940929
  Fax: +91-40-24758499 e-mail: jpmedpub@rediffmail.com
- 1A Indian Mirror Street, Wellington Square, **Kolkata** 700 013,
  Phones: +91-33-22456075, +91-33-22451926, +91-33-30901926 Fax: +91-33-22456075
  e-mail: jpbcal@cal.vsnl.net.in
- 106 Amit Industrial Estate, 61 Dr SS Rao Road, Near MGM Hospital
  Parel, **Mumbai** 400 012, Phones: +91-22-24124863, +91-22-24104532, +91-22-30926896
  Fax: +91-22-24160828 e-mail: jpmedpub@bom7.vsnl.net.in
  e-mail: jpmedpub@bom7.vsnl.net.in
- "KAMALPUSHPA", 38 Reshimbag, Opp. Mohota Science College, Umred Road
  Nagpur 440 009, Phones: +91-712-3945220, +91-712-2704275, Fax: 0712-2704275
  e-mail: jpmednagpur@rediffmail.com

Preventive and Community Dentistry: Clinical Record Book

First Edition: **2006**

ISBN 81-8061-774-2

Typeset at JPBMP typesetting unit
Printed at Gopsons Papers Ltd., A-14, Sector 60, Noida

Preface

" Health is wealth"

Public health is people's health. Oral and dental health is an essential part of overall health.

In order to assess the oral and dental health, it is very important to possess the knowledge of clinical dentistry, epidemiology, behavioural science by the statistics, indices, planning etc.

In order to provide an uniform clinical training programmes in the subject of preventive and community dentistry for BDS students an attempt has been made here to bring out step-by-step clinical procedures in the form of clinical record book. This will help the students to implement their knowledge while examining the patients. It also gives scope to enhance the knowledge of conducting field programmes and understanding the situation existing among the target group of populations like orphanages, old-age homes, primary health centres and similar institutions run by government/private/voluntary organizations.

The main aim of this record book is to enhance the clinical knowledge and organizational abilities of the students to take up public health programmes confidently and complete it successfully.

"Let noble thoughts come to us from every side."
—Upnishad

M Shivakumar

Certificate

This is to certify that the bonafide record of all clinical, field and practical programmes done by Mr/Miss. ____ of ________________ BDS conducted by the Department of Community Dentistry during the academic year ________________________________ at Dental College. His/Her work has been found satisfactory during the period.

Place:

Date:

Professor and Head

Department of Community Dentistry

BDS SYLLABUS FOR CLINICAL TRAINING PROGRAMME IN PREVENTIVE AND COMMUNITY DENTISTRY

The undergraduate student should complete the following clinical and field programme exercises during their postings in the department. Separate postings for students should be arranged in the time table so that the maximum training can be imparted.

I. Clinical Training Programme:

Name of the exercise	No. of cases to be completed
1. Comprehensive oral / dental health planning	10
2. WHO—Oral health assessment form (1997)	10
3. Indices	
A. Dental caries	
DMF – T	10
DMF-S	10
df – t	10
df – s	10
B. Oral hygiene assessment	
Silness and Loe plaque index	5
Greene and Vermillion OHI - S – index	10
C. Gingival and periodontal health assessment	
Russel's periodontal index	10
CPITN index	10
D. Fluorosis index	
Dean's fluorosis index	5
4. Topical fluoride applications:	
a. Sodium fluoride 2%	2
b. Stannous fluoride 8%	2
c. APF solution	2
d. APF gel	2
5. Pit and fissure sealants	2
6. Plaque control programme	5
7. Submission of one model and one chart of public health importance	

II. Field Programmes and Reports

a. Dental camps
b. Visit to water purification plant
c. Visit to primary health centres
d. Visit to slums, villages, etc.
i. Visit to dental clinics
j. Visit to schools
k. Visit to institutions—Handicapped, old age, orphanage, etc.
l. Visit to holistic health centres—Yoga centre, naturopathy centre, music therapy centre, etc.

Contents

CHAPTER ONE

Definitions

HEALTH

WHO Definition: A state of complete physical, mental and social well being and not merely the absence of disease or infirmity.

Talcott Parsons: A state of optimum capacity for the performance of valued task.

Webster's English Dictionary: The soundness or the general wholesomeness of the body.

Perkins: A state of relative equilibrium of body, form and function which results from its successful dynamic equilibrium adjustment of forces to disturb it. It is not passive interplay between body substance and forces impinging upon it but an active response of body forces working towards adjustment.

PUBLIC HEALTH: CHARLES EDWARD A. WINSLOW

It can be defined as the science and art of preventing disease, prolonging life and promoting health and efficiency through organized community efforts for sanitation of environment, control of communicable infections, education of individuals in personal hygiene, organization of medical and nursing services for early diagnosis and preventive treatment of diseases and development of social machinery to ensure for every individual a standard of living adequate for maintenance of health, so organizing these benefits to enable every citizen to realize his birth right of health and longevity.

DENTAL PUBLIC HEALTH

The science and art of preventing and controlling dental diseases and promoting dental health through organized community efforts.

COMMUNITY

It is defined as the group, small or large living together in such a way that the members share not one or more specific interests but rather the basic conditions of common life.

COMMUNITY DENTISTRY

Lars Granath and William D. Mc.Hugh: It is that branch of dentistry which is practiced in relation to population and groups, which derive from epidemiology an awareness of service required and which include the development of technique necessary to organize the application of these services for the benefit of the population.

It is also defined as the field concerned with the study of dental and oral health diseases in the population of a defined community.

COMMUNITY HEALTH

Defined as including all the personal health and environmental services in any human community, irrespective of whether such services were public or private ones.

PREVENTIVE DENTISTRY

It can be defined as a science and art of promoting and preventing the onset of oral and dental diseases and treatment of these diseases in their early stages and prolonging the life by promoting dental or oral health as well as physical and mental health and efficiency of the individuals, families, groups and communities.

Blackerby: It is defined as the efforts made to maintain normal development and physiological functions to prevent diseases of mouth and adjacent parts.

Brauer: Prevention as it applies to the dentistry involves the mechanisms that are employed to combat or intercept dental and systemic diseases which tend to destroy the functions of oral tissues.

PREVENTIVE MEDICINE

Defined as the organized activities of the community to prevent the occurrence as well as progression of the disease and disability, mental and physical and the timely application of all the means to promote the health of the individual and of the community as a whole including prophylaxis, health education and similar work done by a good doctor in looking after individual and family.

SOCIAL MEDICINE

The study of man as a social being in the total environment. It is concerned with the health of groups of individual and individuals within the groups to create, promote, preserve, maintain optimum health.

COMMUNITY MEDICINE

Deals with the population and comprises those doctors who try to measure the needs of the people both sick and well, who plan and administer services to meet those needs and those who are engaged in research and teaching in the field.

COMMUNITY DIAGNOSIS

Refers to the identification and quantification of health problems in a community in terms of mortality and morbidity rates and ratios and the identification of these correlates for the purpose of defining those individuals or groups at risk or those in need of pulp care.

EPIDEMIOLOGY

Parkin (1873): As the branch of medical science which deals with the treatment of epidemics.

Englander (1962): The study of those factors which influence the occurrence and distribution of health, disease, defect, disability and death in population.

John M.Last (1988): The study of the distribution and determinants of health related state and events in specified population and the application of the study to the control of health problems.

Greenwood (1934): The study of disease, any disease as a mass phenomenon.

Macmohan and Pugh (1960): The study of distribution and determinants of disease frequency in man.

EPIDEMIC

The unusual occurrence in a community or region of disease, specific health related behaviour or other health related events clearly in excess of expected occurrence.

ENDEMIC

It refers to the constant presence of a disease or infectious agents within a geographic area or population group without importation from outside.

PANDEMIC

Disease usually affecting a large proportion of population occurring over a wide geographic area.

1. HEALTH EDUCATION

WHO (1969): To persuade people as to adopt and sustain healthy life practices, to use judiciously and wisely the health services available to them, to take their own decision both individually and collectively to improve their status and environment.

2. HEALTH EDUCATION

National conference on preventive medicine USA is defined as the process which informs, motivates and helps people to adopt and maintain healthy practices and lifestyles, advocates environmental changes as needed to facilitate this goal and conducts professional training and research to the same end.

INDEX

Defined as a numerical value describing the relative status of a population on a graduated scale with definite upper and lower limits which is designed to permit and facilitate comparison with other population classified by the same criteria and methods.

SURVEY

It is the investigation where information is systematically collected but in which experimental method is not used. Survey may be descriptive or analytical.

BIOSTATISTICS

It is the method of collecting, organizing, analyzing, tabulating and interpreting of data related to living organisms and human beings.

PLANNING

EC Banfield: A plan is a decision about the course of action. It is the process of preparing a set of decisions for action in the future and must proceed for the development and change in an organization.

EVALUATION

Is defined as the judgement of merit or worth about a particular person, place or thing. It is the collection and analysis of information to determine the programme performance.

WORLD HEALTH ORGANIZATION

It was established in the year 1948 for the purpose of cooperation among themselves and with others to promote the health of the people. Defined by its constitution as the directing and coordination authority on oral health work. It aims in the attainment by all the people of the highest possible level of health.

COMPREHENSIVE DENTAL CARE

It is the meeting of accumulated dental needs at the time a population or group is taken into the program and the detection and correction of new increments of dental disease on a semiannual or other periodic basis.

INCREMENTAL DENTAL CARE

It is defined as a periodic care so spaced that increments of dental diseases are treated at the earliest time consistent with proper diagnosis and operating efficiency in such a way that there is no accumulation of dental needs beyond the minimum.

VOLUNTARY ORGANIZATIONS

Defined as an organization that is administered by an autonomous board which holds meetings, collects funds for its support chiefly from private sectors and expends money with or without paid workers in conducting a programme directed primarily to furthering the public health by providing health education by advancing research or legislation for health or combination of these activities.

Community dentistry has two aspects:

1. Community diagnosis
2. Community treatment.

COMMUNITY DIAGNOSIS

It is a systematic study of community dental and oral health status through epidemiological surveys.

The following data should be collected:

1. Demographic pattern of the community.
2. Socioeconomic conditions of the people.
3. Incidence and prevalence rate of dental and oral diseases.
4. Identification of dental and oral health problems and treatment needs.
5. Identification of high risk and vulnerable group of people.
6. Identification of resources in the community.

COMMUNITY TREATMENT

It aims at planning the oral health programmes and schemes for carrying out oral health and other services required to solve community oral health and other problems. Importance should be given to the FELT NEEDS of the community.

WHAT IS COMMUNITY ORAL HEALTH ?

Community oral health is the organization of an array of promotive, preventive and curative oral health services required at individual and community level for the people living in a community.

DENTAL PUBLIC HEALTH

The American Board of Dental Public Health modified Winslow's definition of public health as the science and art of preventing and controlling dental diseases and promoting dental health through organized community efforts.

It is that form of dental practice that serves the community as a patient rather than an individual. It is concerned with dental health education of public, with research and the application of findings of research, with administration of dental care programme for groups and with prevention and control of dental diseases through a community approach.

THE SCIENCE OF DENTAL PUBLIC HEALTH

It is the concept that oral health service should be aimed at the community level rather than the individual patient level with scientific approach.

It renders the application of principles of Epidemiology, Health Administration, Dental Health Education, Biostatistics, Behavioural Science and Sociology.

THE ART OF DENTAL PUBLIC HEALTH

Applying only scientific principles and arriving at community diagnosis is not sufficient for successful community treatment. The art of dental public health has to be developed. The essential features of the art of community health are:

1. To give priority for the FELT NEEDS
2. To establish co-operation between the health care beneficiaries and providers
3. To utilize all the existing resources with maximum efficiency
4. To establish easy access to health services
5. To give priority to high risk and vulnerable group of people
6. To make health services available and affordable to all
7. To provide comprehensive dental health care.

OBJECTIVES OF COMMUNITY DENTISTRY

1. Health promotion for the entire population.
2. The detection and eradication or control of those factors operating in the community which are imminent to oral health and community well-being.
3. To assess the needs of dental care of the community.
4. Determination of procedures and statement of objectives.
5. Determination of available resources for programme implementation.
6. Improvement of community oral health by:
   a. Implementing effective preventive and therapeutic measures.
   b. Deploying the available resources to meet the needs on the basis of priority.
   c. The measurement of effectiveness of present services and planning of new services.
   d. The co-ordination and integration of dental services and health services.
7. Providing treatment services to persons who do not have easy access to general practitioner.
8. Establishment and maintenance of community laboratories.
9. Co-ordination and participation in the teaching of dental public health and in preventive practices to students, teachers, health educators, dieticians, doctors and nurses.

CHAPTER TWO

Comprehensive Dental Health Care

"It is the complete oral health treatment planning for an individual or a group so that the goal of total oral health is achieved."

DEFINITION

It is a coordinated inter disciplinary approach of providing preventive and therapeutic care followed by maintenance care according to the individuals physical, mental and socio-economic status.

The candidates should be able to plan comprehensive treatment for the individuals or for groups.

Under the guidance of teachers the students must use the specific proforma, should be able to express their views about positive upgrading of oral health status.

1. The personal history details are taken. The chief complaint is noted.
2. The patient is examined for general and dental health status. Clinical findings are noted.
3. The treatment priorities are to be listed out and the levels of prevention for each treatment has to be noted.
4. Lastly the goal which the dental surgeon wants to achieve must be mentioned. For example:
   - Relief from pain
   - Improvement of masticatory efficiency
   - Phonetics—improvements
   - Aesthetics—improvements
   - Social acceptance
   - Social utility of the individual
   - Psychosocial adjustment of the patient.

COMPREHENSIVE DENTAL HEALTH CARE

Case No.: Date:

OP No.:

PERSONAL DATA (BLOCK LETTERS):

Name:

Age:

Gender:

Date and place of birth:

Address:

Phone No:

Religion:

Education:

Occupation:

Income:

Marital Status:

CHIEF COMPLAINTS:

HISTORY OF PRESENT ILLNESS:

PAST DENTAL HISTORY:

MEDICAL HISTORY:

FAMILY HISTORY:

PERSONAL HISTORY:

i. Habits:
   a. Smoking : type / number / frequency / duration
   b. Tobacco chewing : type / frequency / duration
   c. Pan masala / arecanut:
   d. alcohol consumption : type / frequency / duration / quantity

ii. Oral Hygiene Practice:
   a. Type of cleaning : brush / finger / stick / any other ———.
   b. Method of cleaning : vertical / horizontal / circular
   c. Materials used : tooth paste / powder / charcoal / sand / brick powder / salt / any other ——————.
   d. Frequency of cleaning / brushing : once / twice / thrice – a day
   e. Time of brushing : before meal / after meal
   f. Duration of brushing : How long? (time)
   g. Frequency of changing toothbrushes : 3 months / 6 months / 1 year / any other ——
   h. Any other oral hygiene aids used : flossing / interdental brushing / oral mouth rinses / any other ————

iii. Nutritional Status:
   a. Dietary habits: veg / non-veg. / mixed
   b. Source of water
   c. Sugar consumption (per day)
      i. Type
      ii. Frequency—number of times
      iii. Time of intake—with-meals / in-between meals
      iv. Form and consistency—solid / liquid / sticky / nonsticky

GENERAL EXAMINATION:

Height:

Weight:

Gait:

Body type (built):

Posture:

Hands:__________________ Nails: __________________

Physiologic Examination:

a. Speech:

b. Respiration:

c. Swallowing:

Vital Signs:

a. Blood pressure:

b. Pulse rate:

c. Respiratory rate:

d. Temperature:

EXTRAORAL EXAMINATION:

Face and skull:

Face:

a. Symmetry: symmetrical / asymmetrical

b. Profile: convex / concave / straight

c. Lymph nodes:

d. TMJ:

e. Skin:

f. Eyes:

g. Nose:

h. Lips: competent / incompetent

i. Ears:

Skull:

a. Scalp:

b. Hair:

c. Shape of head:

INTRAORAL EXAMINATION

Breath:

Soft Tissue Examination:

a. Buccal mucosa and labial mucosa:

b. Tongue:

c. Floor of the mouth:

d. Palate:

e. Frenum:

f. Salivary gland opening:

g. Tonsils and uvula:

h. Gingiva:

i. Saliva:

Hard Tissue Examination:

a. Type of dentition: Deciduous / mixed / permanent

b. Teeth present:

c. Teeth absent and reasons for loss of teeth:

d. Dental caries:

e. Restored teeth:

f. Any prosthesis:

g. Wasting diseases:

h. Enamel hypoplasia:

i. Supernumerary teeth:

j. Malposition:

k. Occlusion:

l. Occlusal traumatism:

m. Fractured:

n. Stains: extrinsic / intrinsic:

o. Mobility:

p. Any other anomaly:

PROVISIONAL DIAGNOSIS:

RECOMMENDED INVESTIGATIONS:

a. Radiographs:

b. Laboratory Investigations:

DIAGNOSIS:

COMPREHENSIVE TREATMENT PLAN:

CHAPTER THREE

WHO: Oral Health Assessment Form (1997)

Country..

Leave blank (1) ☐☐☐☐ (4) Year Month (5) ☐☐☐☐ (8) Day (9) ☐☐ (10) Identification number (11) ☐☐☐☐ (14) Examiner ☐ (15) Original/duplicate ☐ (16)

General Information

Name...

Date of birth (Year Month) (17) ☐☐☐☐ (20)

Age in years (21) ☐☐ (22)

Sex (M = 1, F = 2) ☐ (23)

Ethnic group ☐ (24)

Occupation ☐ (25)

Geographical location (26) ☐☐ (27)

Location type ☐ (28)
1 = Urban
2 = Periurban
3 = Rural

Other Data (specially and provide codes)

.... ☐ (29)

.... ☐ (30)

Contraindication to examination
Reason : .... ☐ (31)

.... 0 = No
1 = Yes

Clinical Assessment

EXTRAORAL EXAMINATION

0 = Normal extraoral appearance
1 = Ulceration, sores, erosions, fissures (head, neck, limbs)
2 = Ulceration, sores, erosions, fissures (nose cheeks, limbs)
3 = Ulceration, sores, erosions, fissures (commissures)
4 = Ulceration, sores, erosions, fissures (vermillion border)
5 = Cancrum oris
6 = Abnormalities of upper and lower lips
7 = Enlarged lymph nodes (head, neck)
8 = Other swellings of face and jaws
9 = Not recorded

☐ (32)

TEMPOROMANDIBULAR JOINT ASSESSMENT

SYMPTOMS
0 = No
1 = Yes
9 = Not recorded

☐ (33)

SIGNS
0 = No
1 = Yes
9 = Not recorded

Clicking ☐ (34)
Tenderness (on palpation) ☐ (35)
Reduced jaw mobility (>30 mm opening) ☐ (36)

Oral Mucosa

Condition

0 = No abnormal condition
1 = Malignant tumor (oral cancer)
2 = Leukoplakia
3 = Lichen planus
4 = Ulceration (aphthous, herpetic, traumatic)
5 = Acute necrotizing gingivitis
6 = Candidiasis
7 = Abscess
8 = Other condition (specify if possible)
9 = Not recorded

(37) ☐ ☐ (40)
(38) ☐ ☐ (41)
(39) ☐ ☐ (42)

Location

0 = Vermillion
1 = Commissures
2 = Lips
3 = Sulci
4 = Buccal mucosa
5 = Floor of mouth
6 = Tongue
7 = Hard and / or soft palate
8 = Alveolar ridge / gingiva
9 = Not recorded

Enamel Opacities / Hypoplasia
Permanent teeth

0 = Normal
1 = Demarcated opacity
2 = Diffuse opacity
3 = Hypoplasia
4 = Other defects
5 = Demarcated and diffuse opacities
6 = Demarcated opacity and hypoplasia
7 = All three conditions
9 = Not recorded

14 13 12 11 21 22 23 24
(43) ☐☐☐☐☐☐☐☐ (50)
(51) ☐ ☐ (52)
46 36

Dental Fluorosis

0 = Normal
1 = Questionable
2 = Very mild
3 = Mild
4 = Moderate
5 = Severe
8 = Excluded
9 = Not recorded

☐ (53)

Community Periodontal Index (CPI)

0 = Healthy
1 = Bleeding
2 = Calculus
3 = Pocket 4-5 mm (black on probe Partially visible)
4 = Pocket 6 mm or more (black band on probe not visible
x = Excluded sextant
9 = Not recorded
* Not recorded under 15 years of age

17/16 11 26/27
(54) ☐☐☐ (56)
(57) ☐☐☐ (59)
47/46 31 36/37

Loss of Attachment

0 = 0-3 mm
1 = 4-5 mm (cemantoenamel junction (CEJ) within black band
2 = 6-8 mm (CEJ between upper limit of black band and 8.5-mmrimg)
3 = 9-11 mm (CEJ between 8.5-mm and 11.5-mm rings)
4 = 12 mm or more (CEJ beyond 11.5-mm ring)
x = Excluded sextant
9 = Not recorded
* Not recorded under 15 years of age

17/16 11 26/27
(54) ☐☐☐ (56)
(57) ☐☐☐ (59)
47/46 31 36/37

DENTITION STATUS AND TREATMENT NEED

Identification number ☐☐☐☐

				55	54	53	52	51	61	62	63	64	65			
	18	17	16	15	14	13	12	11	21	22	23	24	25	26	27	28
Crown (66)																(82)
Root (82)																(97)
Treatment (98)																(113)

				85	84	83	82	81	71	72	73	74	75			
	48	47	46	45	44	43	42	41	31	32	33	34	35	36	37	38
Crown (114)																(129)
Root (130)																(145)
Treatment (146)																(161)

Primary teeth Crown	Permanent teeth Crown	Permanent teeth Root	STATUS
A	0	0	Sound
B	1	1	Decayed
C	2	2	Filled, no decay
D	3	3	Filled, no decay
E	4	–	Missing, as a result of caries
–	5	–	Miising, any other reason
F	6	–	Fissure sealent
G	7	7	Bridge abutment, special crown or veneer/implant
I	8	8	Unrupted tooth (crown)/unexpected root
T	T	–	Trauma (fracture)
–	9	9	Not recorded

TREATMENT

0 = None
P = Preventive, caries arresting care
F = Fissure Sealent
1 = One surface filling
2 = Two or more surface Fillings
3 = Crwon for any reason
4 = Veneer or laminate
5 = Pulp care and restoration
6 = Extraction
7 = Need for other care (specify)....................
8 = Need for other care (specify)
9 = Not recorded

Prosthetics Status

Upper lower

(162) ☐☐ (163)

0 = No prosthetics
1 = Bridge
2 = More than one bridge
3 = Partial denture
4 = Bothe bridge(s) and partialdenture(s)
5 = Full removable denture
9 = Not recorded

Prosthetics Need

Upper lower

(164) ☐☐ (165)

0 = No prosthesis needed
1 = Need for one-unit prosthesis
2 = Need for multi-unit prosthesis
3 = Need for a combination of one and/or multi-unit prostheses
4 = Need for full prosthesis (replacement of all teeth)
9 = Not recorded

DENTOFACIAL ANOMALIES

DEFINITION

(166) ☐☐ (167) Missing incisor, canine and premolar teeth - maxillary and mandibular - enter number of teeth

SPACE

☐ (168) Crowding in the incisal segments in mm
0 = No crowding
1 = One segment crowded
2 = Two segment crowded

☐ (169) Spacing in the incisal segments in mm
0 = No spacing
1 = One spaced
2 = Two segment spaced

☐ (170) Diastema in mm

☐ (171) Largest anterior maxillary irregularity

☐ (172) Largest anterior mandibular irregularity

OCCLUSION

☐ (173) Anterior maxillary overjet in mm

☐ (174) Anterior mandibular overjet in mm

☐ (175) Vertical anterior openbite in mm

☐ (176) Antero-posterior molar relation
0 = Normal
1 = Half cusp
2 = Full cusp

NEED FOR IMMEDIATE CARE AND REFERRAL

Life threatening condition ☐ (129)
Plain or infection ☐ (145)
Other condition (specify)..................... ☐ (161)

0 = Absent
1 = Present
9 = Not recorded

Referral ☐ (180)
0 = No
1 = Yes
9 = Not recorded

NOTES

CHAPTER FOUR

Dental Indices in Dental Epidemiological Surveys

WHAT IS DENTAL INDEX?

An index has been defined by Russel as "a numerical value describing the relative status of a population on a graduated scale with definite upper and lower limits, which is designed to permit and facilitate comparison with other populations classified by the same criteria and methods."

An index is an expression of clinical observations in numerical values.

Ideal Requirements of an Index

1. The examiner should be able to carry the rules of the index in his mind.
2. The index should be reasonably easy to apply so that there is no undue loss of time during field examinations.
3. The criteria for the index should be clear and unambiguous
4. **Validity:** The index must measure what is intended to measure, so it should correspond with clinical stages of the disease under study at each point.
5. **Reliability and reproducibility:** The index should be reliable and reproducible means the ability of the same or different examiners to interpret and use the index in the same way.
6. **Quantifiability:** The index should be amenable to statistical analysis.
7. **Sensitivity:** The index should be able to detect reasonably small shifts in either direction in the group condition.
8. **Acceptability:** An index should be universally acceptable.
9. **Cost and material:** Require minimal equipment and expenditure.
10. **Comfort:** Not to cause any discomfort to the patient.

WHAT ARE THE USES OF DENTAL INDICES?

A. In Individual oral health assessment scores

B. In clinical trials

C. In community health epidemiologic surveys.

Individual Oral Health Assessment Score

Purpose

In clinical practice an index is used to record details of an individual patient which can be used for education, motivation, evaluation and treatment planning.

Uses

i. Provides individual assessment to help a patient recognise an oral and dental problem.

ii. Reveals the degree of effectiveness of present oral hygiene practices.

iii. Motivates the person in preventive and professional care for the elimination and control of dental diseases.

iv. Evaluates the success of individual and professional treatment over a period of time by comparing index scores.

Clinical Trial

Purpose

A clinical trial is planned for the determination of the effect of an agent or procedure on the progression, control and prevention of dental disease. The trial is conducted by comparing an experimental group with a control group that is similar to the experimental group in every way except for the variable being studied.

Uses

i. Determines baseline data before experimental factors are introduced.

ii. Measures the effectiveness of specific agents for the prevention, control, and treatment of oral and dental diseases.

iii. Measures the effectiveness of mechanical devices for personal care such as toothbrushes, interdental cleaning devices and water irrigators.

Community Health Epidemiological Survey

Purpose

The word Epidemiology denotes the study of disease characteristics of populations. An example of an index designed for a survey of population groups is DMF Index. It has been used with populations around the world to determine the extent of dental caries. Such a survey was not designed for evaluation of an individual patient.

Uses

i. Shows the prevalence and incidence of a particular oral and dental disease condition occurring within a given population.
ii. To facilitate comparisons between populations.
iii. To assess the needs of a community
iv. To compare the effects of a community program and evaluates the results.
v. In community health programmes the dental index is employed to provide proof of legitimacy and effectiveness.
vi. Serve as an evaluation mechanism for the profession and public in estimating future needs and evaluation treatment of preventive procedures.

TYPES OF INDICES

a. Simple index
b. Cumulative index.

a. **Simple Index:** Which measures the presence or absence of a condition. For example an index that measures the presence of bacterial plaque without evaluation of its effect on the gingiva.
b. **Cumulative Index**: Which measures all the evidences of a condition past and present. An example is the DMF Index for dental caries. Depending upon the reversible change of disease conditions the simple and cumulative indices are classified into:
   1. **Reversible index:** Indices are used to measure changing conditions that may heal or progress with time, e.g. gingivitis, bacterial plaque. OHI-S, plaque index, GI, PHPI, PMA, gingival bleeding.
   2. **Irreversible index:** Which measures conditions that will not change. These indices are used to measure cumulative conditions. They are extremely valuable in longitudinal studies to determine changes over a specific period of time, e.g. dental caries.

3. **Reversible-irreversible:** Indices are used to measure both reversible and irreversible conditions of a disease, e.g. Russel's periodontal index.

SELECTION OF DENTAL INDICES

This is determined by the following factors:

1. Type of conditions to be assessed
2. Age of the population to be studied.
3. Purpose of the research.

CHAPTER FIVE

Dental Caries Index

The first description of DMF index is usually attributed to Henry Klein, Carrol E Palmer and JW Knutson (1938).

WHAT IS DMFT INDEX?

Definition

DMFT index is a quantitative expression of a person's lifetime caries experience in the permanent teeth.

A DMF index is the sum of decayed (D) missing, extracted because of caries (M) and filled because of caries. (F), permanent teeth (T) or tooth surfaces (S). [Bodecker developed an index to measure dental caries. But it was elaborate, complicated and cannot be used in field work].

The DMF index for permanent teeth is always signified by upper case letters. The equivalent index for primary teeth is the "def" and its modifications, signified by lower case letters.

WHAT IS DMF INDEX ?

DMF is a quantitative expression of caries experience or caries prevalence in the primary teeth. It is the sum of decayed (d) missing due to caries (m) and filled (f) primary teeth (t) or tooth surfaces (s). It is used in the same way as the DMF index. It is introduced by Gruebbel in 1944.

DF index: Is a quantitative expression of a person or group number of decayed and filled permanent teeth / tooth surfaces.

df index: Is a quantitative expression of a child's or group of children's number of decayed and filled primary teeth / tooth surfaces.

def index: Is a quantitative expression of observable caries experience or caries prevalence in the primary dentition. It is the sum of the number of primary teeth or surfaces that are decayed (d), decayed beyond repair, that is those that need to be extracted (e) or filled (f).

USES OF DMF INDEX

A survey using DMF index can provide information of:

a. The number of persons affected by dental caries
b. The number of teeth requiring treatment for the disease (dental caries)
c. The proportion of teeth that have been treated (filled because of dental caries)
d. The proportion of teeth that have been extracted because of dental caries.
e. The DMF statistical data are useful in evaluating and directing dental health programmes.
f. DMF index also provides data useful in assessing the value of various preventive activities, e.g. water fluoridation, topical fluoride application, etc.
g. DMF index helps the governing bodies in assessing the need for additional dental resources and financial support to provide the treatment and preventive measures needed in the community.

LIMITATIONS OF DMF INDEX

1. The DMF values are not related to the number of teeth at risk.
2. The DMF index can be invalid in older adults because teeth can be lost for reasons other than caries.
3. The DMF index can be misleading in children whose teeth have been extracted for orthodontic reasons and also due to trauma, or accidents.
4. The DMF index can overestimate caries experience in teeth with preventive restorations or where treatment services are intense.
5. The DMF cannot be used for root caries.
6. The DMF cannot account for root canal treated teeth.

EXAMINATION CRITERIA AND RULES FOR CODING

Special Rules

1. No tooth should be counted more than once. It is either decayed, missing, filled or sound.
2. D, M and F teeth should be recorded separately since the components of DMF are of great interest.
3. A tooth is considered erupted when the occlusal surface or incisal edge is totally exposed or can be exposed by gently reflecting any overlying gingival tissues with the mirror or explorer.

4. A tooth is considered to be present even though the crown has been destroyed and only the roots are left in the socket.
5. Super numerary teeth are not included.
6. If a primary tooth is retained and its permanent successor is present, classify the permanent tooth.
7. Primary teeth are not included in "DMF" count nor permanent teeth in "def" count. They should be counted separately i.e. permanent teeth in "DMF" and deciduous teeth in "def" indices.
8. A tooth may have several restorations but it should be counted as one filled tooth.
9. WHO modifications of DMF (1986).
   a. All 3rd molars are included.
   b. Temporary restorations are considered as 'D' decayed.
   c. Only caries cavities are considered as 'D', the initial lesions (chalky spots, stained fissures) are not considered as 'D'.
10. Care must be taken to list as missing only those teeth which have been lost due to caries.
    Also include those teeth which are so badly decayed that they are indicated for extraction.
    The following should not be considered as missing:
    i. Unerupted teeth.
    ii. Missing teeth due to accident.
    iii. Congenitally missing teeth.
    iv. Teeth extracted for orthodontic treatment.
11. In deciduous dentition naturally exfoliated teeth should not be taken into consideration.
12. In DMFS and dfs indices, if the anterior tooth is missing due to caries 4 surfaces and if posterior tooth is missing due to caries 5 surfaces should be considered.
13. If there is a filling and carious lesions are present on the same surface that surface is considered as only one surface that too as caries.
14. Sealed tooth with decay is considered as decayed.
15. The DMF index is not designed for use with root caries.

EXCLUSIONS

Excluded Tooth/Tooth Spaces

1. The tooth has been fractured and the fractured portion is treated with a filling, jacket crown, etc.

2. The tooth has root canal filling due to trauma.
3. The tooth has a jacket crown because it is poorly formed tooth, e.g. peg shaped laterals.
4. The tooth has a restoration used as a bridge abutment.
5. A permanent tooth has been removed for orthodontic treatment or for any reason other than caries.(periodontal disease, impaction, etc.)
6. Supernumerary teeth.

CRITERIA FOR DIAGNOSIS AND CODING

Permanent Tooth Present

Code 1: Sound Permanent Tooth

If there is no indication of caries and no fillings, jacket crowns or bridge abutment. Other defects such as hypoplasia, fluorosis, enamel defects may/may not be present. If some surfaces of an apparently sound tooth are obscured by an orthodontic band, assume that the tooth is sound.

Code 2: Filled Permanent Tooth.

When a tooth has been filled permanently because of dental caries.

Note:

1. A tooth that is both filled and decayed is classified as decayed.
2. In any instance where the filling has been dislodged or fractured it is classified as decayed.

Code 3: Decayed Permanent Tooth.

When the following evidence of caries present.

a. **Visual Examination:** Visual evidence of undermined enamel, there must be a definite cavitation with either discolouration (grayish-white undermined enamel) or opacity around the edges or loss of transluscency and in which the explorer tip can penetrate into soft yielding material.
b. Pit and fissures in which the end of explorer catch should be classified as carious only if one of the following criterion is present.
   i. Tactile (perceptible by touch or pertaining to sense of touch), perceptible is that which may be known by sense) evidence of soft carious material at the base of pit.
   ii. Opacity around the edges or an underlying stain typical of dental caries.
   iii. Grayish-white colour spreading from margins of restoration caused by lesions of secondary dental caries.

PRIMARY TEETH PRESENT

Use the same criteria as for classification of permanent tooth present.

Code as follows:

1. Code E: Excluded tooth or tooth space (both primary and permanent dentition).
2. Code PI: Sound primary tooth
3. Code P2: Filled primary tooth
4. Code P3: Carious primary tooth.
5. Code 0: Missing tooth other than caries, code a tooth space as " 0" when there is absence of a tooth is due to one of the following:
   - Primary/permanent tooth missing for any reason other than decay (exfoliation, periodontitis)
   - Primary or permanent tooth is absent,
     - unerupted primary tooth.
     - unerupted permanent tooth
   - Impacted or congenitally missing primary/permanent tooth.
6. Code X: Extracted permanent tooth.
   - Code tooth space as "X"

If according to the age of a person a permanent tooth should be present but in all probability has been extracted because of caries.

Note: i. Ask question regarding extraction

ii. Use clinical judgement for missing.

DMFT AND DMFS

Purpose: To determine dental caries experience past and present for children older than 7 years and upto 12 years of age.

Selection of Teeth or Surfaces

a. DMFT: 12 teeth evaluated (8 primary molars and 4 primary canines)

b. DMFS: 56 surfaces.

primary molars 8 multiplied by 5 surfaces = 40 surfaces.

primary canines 4 multiplied by 4 surfaces = 16 surfaces.

c. A primary molar/canine is presumed missing because of dental caries when it has been lost before the normal exfoliation time.

PROCEDURE

a. Instruments and examination: similar to DMFT

b. Criteria:

d: number of molars and canines that are carious or number of surfaces that are carious.

m: number of primary molars and canines missing because of dental caries.

f: number of permanently filled molars and canines without dental caries.

SCORING

Individual DMF

A 10-year-old boy has all primary molars and canines present.

Examination reveals: d = 2 m = 0 f = 1

dmf = d+ m + f = 2 + 0 + 1 = 3

CARIES INDEX

DMFT, DMFS, dft, dfs, Index

Name: ______________________ Date :__________

Oral Hygiene Habit: __________ Case No.______ Age:_____ Sex:________

Frequency:______________________ Occupation:__________

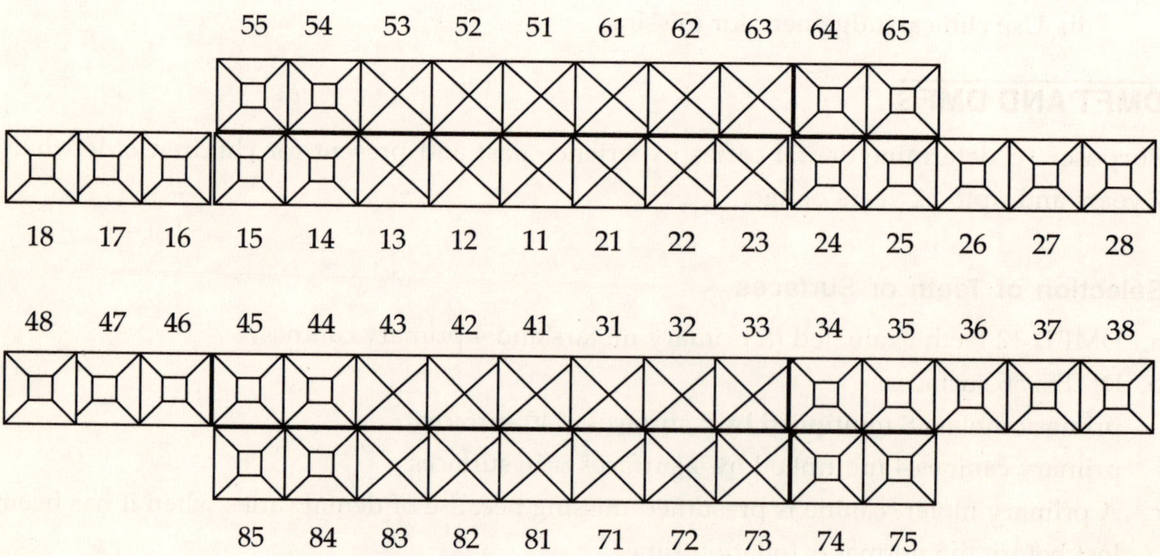

DMFT/dft	DMFS/dfs	
D/d =	D/d =	Decayed
M =	M =	Missing
F/f =	F/f =	Filled
DMFT/dft Score =	DMFS/dfs Score =	

Staff Signature:

Date:

CHAPTER SIX

Oral Hygiene Index: Simplified (Greene and Vermillion–1964)

Greene and Vermillion developed the Oral Hygiene Index (OHI) in 1960 and later simplified in 1964.

WHY IS OHI SIMPLIFIED?

The original method of OHI required the examination of selected 12 tooth surfaces 1 facial and 1 lingual or palatal on each segment, that are covered with the greatest amount of debris plaque or calculus.

Realising that it was neither practical nor necessary to assess 12 tooth surfaces to determine a person's level of oral cleanliness because

1. The length of time required to evaluate debris and calculus.
2. As well as to make subjective decisions on tooth selection. In OHI the examiner has to select the teeth with the most debris or calculus in each segment.
3. Since, the OHI procedure is very much tiring and time consuming may cause loss of interest of examiner and hence not suitable for epidemiological surveys.

Therefore, in 1964 Greene and Vermillion simplified the OHI.

Differences between OHI and OHI-S

	OHI	OHI-S
1. Tooth selection	The examiner has to select the teeth with the most debris or calculus in each segment	OHI-S assesses 6 index teeth one in each segment
2. No. of surfaces	12 surfaces are evaluated	only 6 surfaces are evaluated
3. Scoring	The OHI ranges from 0 to 12.	OHI-S ranges from 0 to 6

Simplified Oral Hygiene Index (OHI-S)

Purpose: To assess oral cleanliness by estimating the tooth surface covered with debris/ calculus to know the oral hygiene status of individual.

Selection of Teeth and Surfaces

1. Divide the dentition into segments,
   a. Anterior canine to canine
   b. Posterior segment begins distal to the second premolar.

   Score only 1st fully-erupted permanent teeth distal to 2nd premolars in each posterior segment and maxillary right and mandibular left central incisors.

   Facial surfaces of the maxillary right and mandibular left central incisors are used. When either is missing then opposite central incisor is scored

2. **Index teeth**

6 1	6
6	1 6

   A tooth is considered fully erupted when it has reached the occlusal plane. IIIrd molars are included only when it has reached occlusal plane fully-erupted and functional.

   Note: Exclusion:
   1. IIIrd molars
   2. Teeth with full crown restorations
   3. Tooth reduced in height because of dental caries or trauma.

3. **Tooth surfaces:**

   Lingual surfaces of 36, 46 and buccal surfaces of 16, 26 and labial surfaces of 11,31.

4. **Extent:**

   A score represents half the circumference of the selected tooth includes proximal surfaces to the contact areas.

5. **Components:**

   The OHI-S has two components:
   - Simplified debris index (Dl - S)
   - Simplified calculus index (Cl - S)

   The two scores may be used separately or may be combined for OHI - S

Procedure

a. **Qualification:** At least two of the six possible surfaces must have been examined for an individual score to be expressed.

b. **Evaluation:** Evaluate each segment to record first the debris and then the calculus to avoid accidental removal of debris from the tooth surface.

c. **Sequence:** Proceed in routine order from maxillary right anterior and left segment to mandibular left anterior and right segment.

d. **Record:** Six debris scores.

1. **Oral debris:** Is the soft foreign matter loosely attached to the teeth. It consists of mucin, bacterial plaque, materia alba and food debris. It varies in colour from grayish white to green or orange.
   - **Mucin:** Secretion of the mucous or goblet cells a polysaccharide protein which combine with water forms a solution called mucous contained in saliva.
   - **Bacterial plaque:** Is a dense non mineralized complex mass of bacterial colonies in a gel-like intermicrobial matrix. It adheres firmly to the acquired pellicle and hence to the teeth, calculus, and fixed or removable restorations.
   - **Materia alba:** It is a loosely adherent mass of bacteria and cellular debris that frequently occurs on top of bacteria plaque.
   - **Food debris:** Loose food particles collect above the cervical third and proximal embrasures of the teeth.
2. **Extrinsic stains:** It is a thin layer of foreign matter firmly attached to the surface of the tooth but may be removed by scraping with the tip of an explorer. Colour may range from black to dark brown, green or reddish orange.
3. **Examination:** Run the side of the tip of a probe or an explorer across the tooth surface from incisor or occlusal third to cervical third to assist in estimating the surface area covered by debris.
4. **Criteria:**

   0 = No debris or stains present

   1 = Soft debris covering not more than one third of the tooth surface being examined or the presence of extrinsic stains without debris regardless of surface area covered.

   2 = Soft debris covering more than one third but not more than two third of the exposed tooth surface.

   3 = Soft debris covering more than two-thirds of the exposed tooth surface.

e. **Record six calculus scores:**

Definition of calculus: Oral calculus is a hard deposit of inorganic salt composed primarily of calcium carbonate and phosphate mixed with debris, microorganisms and desquamated epithelial cells.

Supragingival calculus: Is usually white to yellowish brown and is deposited occlusal to the free gingival margin.

Subgingival calculus: Is usually light brown colour because of inclusion of blood pigments and is deposited apical to the free gingival margin on the cervical portion of the tooth.

Use an explorer to supplement visual examination for supragingival calculus deposits. Identify subgingival deposits by exploring and/or probing. Record only definite deposits of hard calculus.

0 = No calculus present

1 = Only supragingival calculus covering not more than 1/3 of the exposed tooth surface.

2 = Supragingival calculus covering more than 1/3 but not more than 2/3 of the exposed tooth surface or the presence of individual flecks of subgingival calculus around the cervical portion of the tooth.

3 = Supragingival calculus covering more than 2/3 of the exposed tooth surface or a continuous band of subgingival calculus around the cervical portion of the tooth.

Scoring

A. Calculation for individual OHI-S

$$\text{Debris index simplified} = \frac{\text{Total debris score}}{\text{No. of tooth surfaces examined}} = \frac{\qquad}{6}$$

$$\text{Calculus index simplified} = \frac{\text{Total calculus score}}{\text{No. of tooth surfaces examined}} = \frac{\qquad}{6}$$

For individual DI-S and CI-S values ranges from 0 to 3.

Simplified Oral Hygiene Index for an individual

OHI-S = DI-S + CI-S

OHI-S values range from 0 to 6

B. Suggested nominal scale:

D I – S and C I – S		***OHI-S***	
Rating	**Scores**	**Rating**	**Scores**
Good	0.1 - 0.6	Good	0.1 - 1.2
Fair	0.7 - 1.8	Fair	1.3 - 3.0
Poor	1.9 - 3.0	Poor	3.1 - 6.0

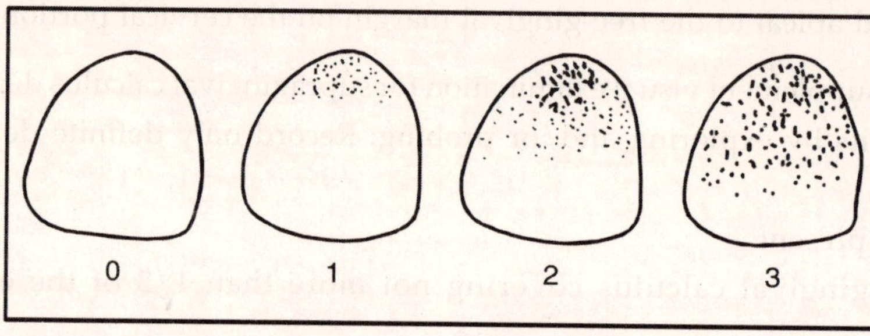

Figure 6.1: Showing scoring of 0 to 3 is based on tooth surfaces covered by debris

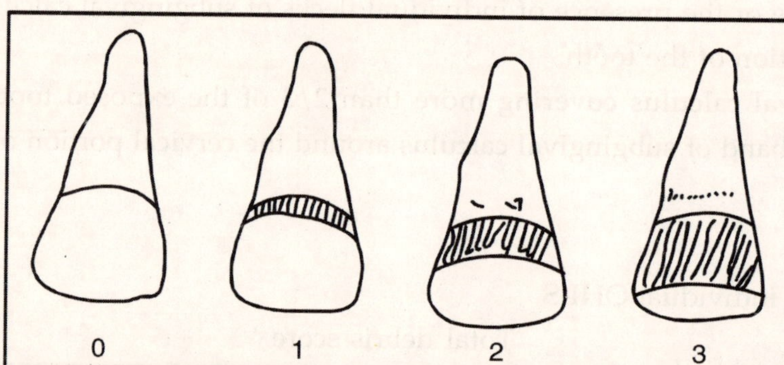

Figure 6.2: Showing scoring of 0 to 3 is based on tooth surfaces covered by calculus

Debris Scores:

16	11	26
46	31	36

Debris Index – S = $\frac{\quad}{6}$ =

Calculus Scores:-

16	11	26
46	31	36

Calculus Index – S = $\frac{\quad}{6}$ =

Calculation for Individual OHI-S

$$\text{Debris Index-S} = \frac{\text{Total debris scores}}{\text{Number of surfaces}} = \frac{\qquad}{6}$$

$$\text{Calculus Index-S} = \frac{\text{Total calculus scores}}{\text{Number of surfaces}} = \frac{\qquad}{6}$$

Greene and Vermillion Oral Hygiene Index — Simplified (OHI-S)

Name:______________________________ Date________________

Oral Hygiene Habit: Case No.______________ Age:____________ Sex:__________

Frequency:____________ Occupation: ______________________________

Debris Index-Simplified: (DI-S)

16	11	26
46	31	36

Debris Index – S = $\frac{\quad}{6}$ =

Calculus Index-Simplified: (CI-S)

16	11	26
46	31	36

Calculus Index – S = $\frac{\quad}{6}$ =

OHI(S) = DI-S + CI-S

Staff Signature:

Date:

CHAPTERSEVEN

Plaque Index (Silness and Loe–1964)

PURPOSE

To assess the thickness of plaque at the gingival area

SELECTION OF TEETH

Scoring is done on	16	22	24
	44	42	36

AREAS EXAMINED

Four gingival areas—facial, lingual, mesial and distal are examined systematically for index tooth.

OR

Examine on the facial, mesial and lingual areas assign double score for the mesial reading 7 divide the total by 4.

PROCEDURE

1. Dry the teeth and visual examination is done under adequate light using mouth mirror and probe.
2. Evaluate the bacterial plaque only on the cervical 3rd, pay no attention to plaque on the middle and occlusal 3rd.
3. Probe to test the surface when no plaque is visible. Pass the probe or explorer across the tooth surface in the cervical 3rd, and near the entrance to the sulcus. When no plaque adheres to the probe tip the area is scored 0. If plaque adheres then a score 1 is assigned.
4. Use disclosing solution if necessary to assist evaluation of 0/1 scores.

5. When plaque index is used in conjunction with gingival index, the gingival index must be completed first because the disclosing agent will mask the gingival characteristics.
6. Include the plaque on the surface of calculus and on restorations in the cervical 3rd in evaluation.

CRITERIA FOR SCORING

0 - No plaque

1 - A thin film of plaque adhering to free gingival margin and adjacent area of the tooth.

2- Moderate accumulation of soft deposits within the gingival pocket that can be seen with naked eye or on tooth and gingival margin.

3- Abundance of soft matter within gingival pocket, on the tooth and gingival margin.

SCORING

A. Plaque index for an area; each of the areas (mesial, lingual and buccal) are assigned Scores from 0 to 3.

B. Plaque index for a tooth: scores of each area are totalled and divided by 4.

C. Plaque index for an individual: add the scores for each tooth and divide by the number of teeth examined.

D. Suggested nominal scale for patient reference

RATING	SCORES
Excellent	0
Good	0.1-0.9
Fair	1.0-1.9
Poor	2.0-3.0

SILNESS AND LOE (1964) PLAQUE INDEX

Name:____________________________ Date:______________

Oral Hygiene Habit:______________ Case No. Age: Sex:

Frequency:____________________________ Occupation:______________

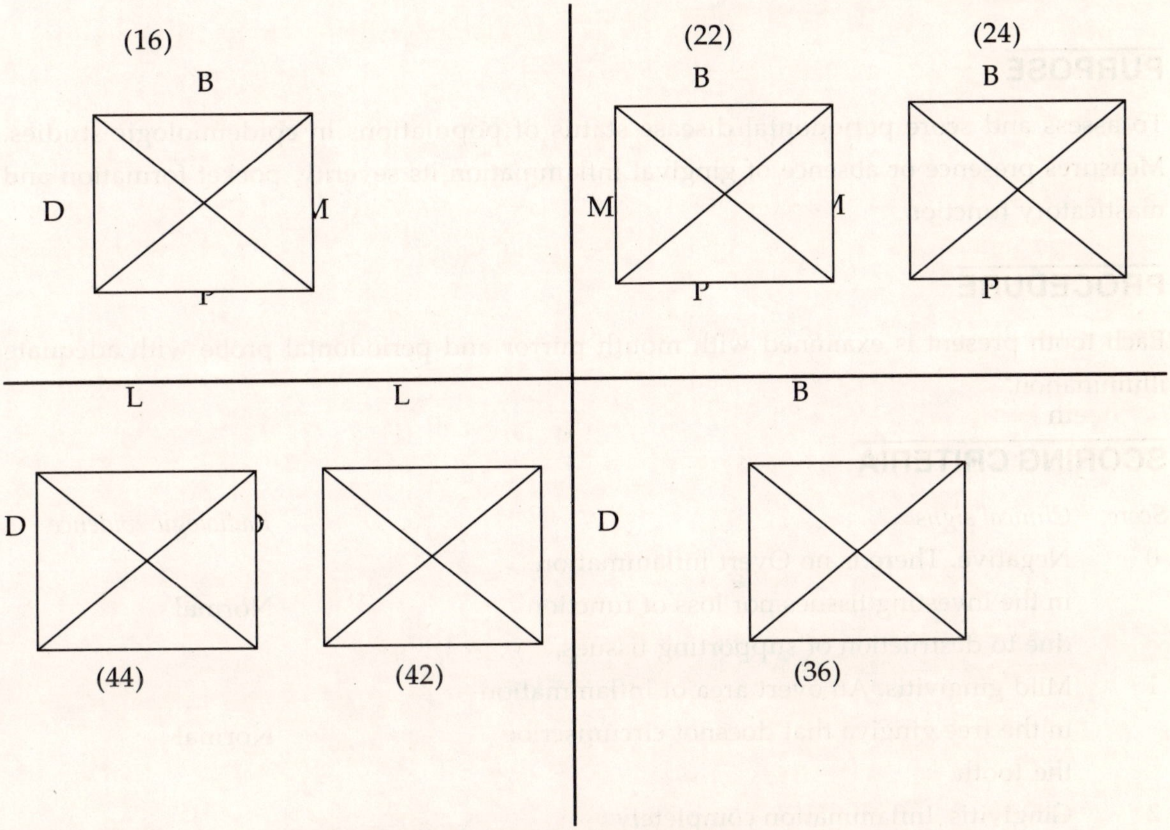

$$\text{Plaque Index} = \frac{\text{Sum of all individual plaque scores}}{\text{Total no. of surfaces examined}} = \frac{\quad}{24} =$$

Staff Signature

Date:

CHAPTER EIGHT

Periodontal Index (PI)–Russell

PURPOSE

To assess and score periodontal disease status of populations in epidemiologic studies. Measures presence or absence of gingival inflammation its severity, pocket formation and masticatory function.

PROCEDURE

Each tooth present is examined with mouth mirror and periodontal probe with adequate illumination.

SCORING CRITERIA

Score	*Clinical signs*	*Radiologic evidence*
0	Negative. There is no Overt inflammation in the investing tissues nor loss of function due to destruction of supporting tissues.	Normal
1	Mild gingivitis. An overt area of inflammation in the free gingiva that doesnot circumscribe the tooth.	Normal
2	Gingivitis. Inflammation completely circumscribes the tooth but no apparent break in the epithelial attachment.	Normal
4	————	Radiograph shows notch like resorption of the crest of alveolar bone.

6	Gingivitis with pocket formation. The epithelial attachment is broken and pocket is formed. No interference with the normal masticatory function tooth is firm and not drifted.	Horizontal bone loss involving the entire alveolar and crest up to half of the root length.
8	Advanced destruction with loss of masticatory function. The tooth may be loose, may be drifted, may sound dull on percussion with the metallic instrument, may be depressable in the socket.	Advanced bone loss involving more than one half of length of the root or a definite infrabony pocket with widening of periodontal space. There may be root resorption or rarefaction at the apex.

SCORING:

A. Each Tooth is assigned a score from 0 to 8 (When in doubt assign a lesser score)

B. Add scores of each tooth and divide by the number of teeth present or examined to obtain the individual score.

$$\text{Periodontal index score per person} = \frac{\text{Sum of individual scores}}{\text{Number of teeth present}}$$

C. Periodontal index group score – Total the individual score and divide by the number of individual examined.

D. Interpretation of the score results:

Group PI score	*Clinical condition*	*Stage of the disease*
0 to 0.2	Clinically normal supportive tissues	
0.3 to 0.9	Simple gingivitis	Reversible
1.0 to 1.9	Beginning of the destructive periodontal disease	Reversible
2.0 to 4.0	Established destructive periodontal disease	Irreversible
4.1 to 8.0	Terminal disease	Irreversible

(Score 2 to 8, clinical condition can certainly be improved with appropriate treatment planning by the periodontist)

RUSSELL'S PERIODONTAL INDEX (PI)

Name:____________________ Date:__________

Oral hygiene habit:__________ Case No.____ Age:____ Sex:____

Frequency:__________ Occupation:__________

18	17	16	15	14	13	12	11	21	22	23	24	25	26	27	28
48	47	46	45	44	43	42	41	31	32	33	34	35	36	37	38

Total score =

Total no. of teeth examined = **P.I. =**

Periodontal health condition = __________

Name:____________________ **Date:**__________

Oral hygiene habit: __________ **Case No.**____ **Age:**____ **Sex:**____

Frequency:__________ **Occupation:** __________

18	17	16	15	14	13	12	11	21	22	23	24	25	26	27	28
48	47	46	45	44	43	42	41	31	32	33	34	35	36	37	38

Total score =

Total no. of teeth examined = **P.I. =**

Periodontal health condition =

CHAPTER NINE

Community Periodontal Index of Treatment Needs (CPITN)

The CPITN was developed in colloboration between the FDI and the oral health unit of the WHO in 1982. A description of the methodology has been published by AINAMO and his associates.

PURPOSE

To screen and monitor individual or group periodontal treatment needs.

SELECTION OF TEETH

1. The Periodontal treatment needs are recorded for sextants, i.e. 6th of the dentition.
2. III Molars are not included except when they are functioning in the place of II Molars.
3. The sextants containing the following teeth.

17-14	13-23	24-27
47-44	43-33	34-37

4. The treatment need in a sextant is recorded only when 2 or more teeth are present and not indicated for extraction.

USE OF INDEX TEETH

In epidemiological surveys assessing periodontal treatment needs of a population the recordings per sextant are based on findings from specified index teeth.

ADULTS: (20 years and above).

1. The index teeth to be examined are

17/16	11	26/27
47/46	31	36/37

2. Although 10 index teeth are examined only 6 recordings, one relating to each sextant are made.
3. When both or one of the designated molar teeth are present, the worst finding from these surfaces is recorded for the sextant.
4. If no index teeth are present in a sextant qualifying for examination, all the remaining teeth in that sextant are examined.

CHILDREN AND ADOLESCENTS (7-19 YEARS)

1. Divide the dentition into sextants as mentioned above.
2. Index teeth

16	11	26
26	31	36

3. When the designated tooth is missing, the sextant is recorded as missing and marked as "X".

PROCEDURE

1. Objectives: A tooth is probed to determine.
   i. Pocket depth
   ii. Presence of calculus
   iii. Bleeding response
2. Probing force: It can be divided into
   i. a working component—to determine pocket depth
   ii. a sensing component—to detect subgingival calculus.

   Use force no greater than 25 grams to reveal disease without causing discomfort to the patient.
3. When inserting the probe into a pocket the ball point should follow the anatomic configuration of the root surface along the long axis of tooth.
4. For sensing subgingival calculus, the lightest possible force which allows movement of the probe a ball point along the tooth surface is used. Observe colour coded area for prompt identification of pocket depth below 3.5 mm, between 3.5 and 5.5 mm (within the colour coded zone) and above the 5.5 mm to facilitate classification.

CRITERIA

Code 0: Healthy periodontium

Code 1: Bleeding observed after gentle probing

Code 2: Calculus felt on probing or defective margin of filling or crown.

Code 3: Pocket depth between 3.5 and 5.5 mm where the black band is visible.

Code 4: Pocket depth more than 5.5 mm where the black band is not visible.

SCORING

A. Periodontal treatment needs scale

Patients are classified (0,I, II, III) in treatment needs according to the highest code recorded during examination.

0: No need for treatment (code 0)

I: Oral hygiene instructions (code 1)

II: Oral hygiene instructions, scaling and root planing including correction of plaque retentive margins of fillings and crowns (code 2 and 3).

III: Oral hygiene instructions, scaling and complex periodontal treatment, surgical intervention (code 4)

B. CPITN for an individual and group

1. The CPITN provides percentage of subjects having healthy periodontal tissues, bleeding only, bleeding with presence of calculus and with periodontal pockets.

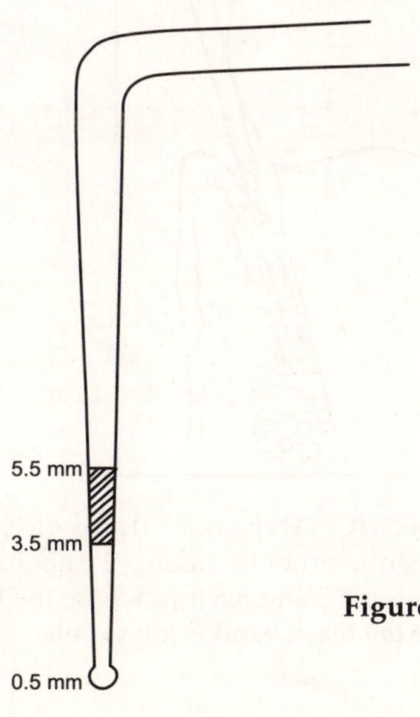

Figure 9.1: CPITN—E probe for an epidemiological study (with one black band 3.5 – 5.5 mm)

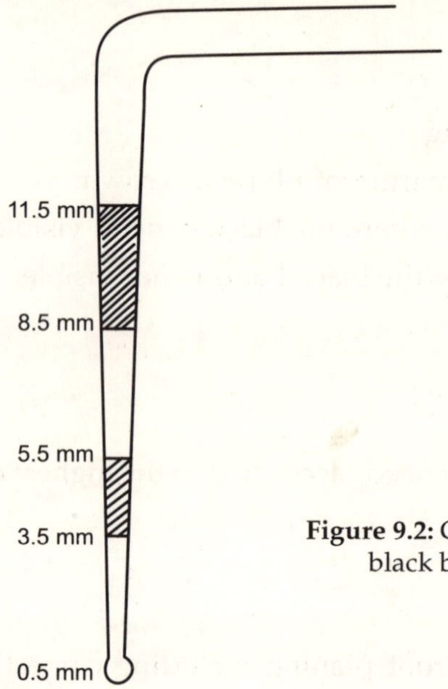

Figure 9.2: CPITN–C probe for clinical study (with two black bands 3.5 – 5.5 mm and 8.5 – 11.5 mm)

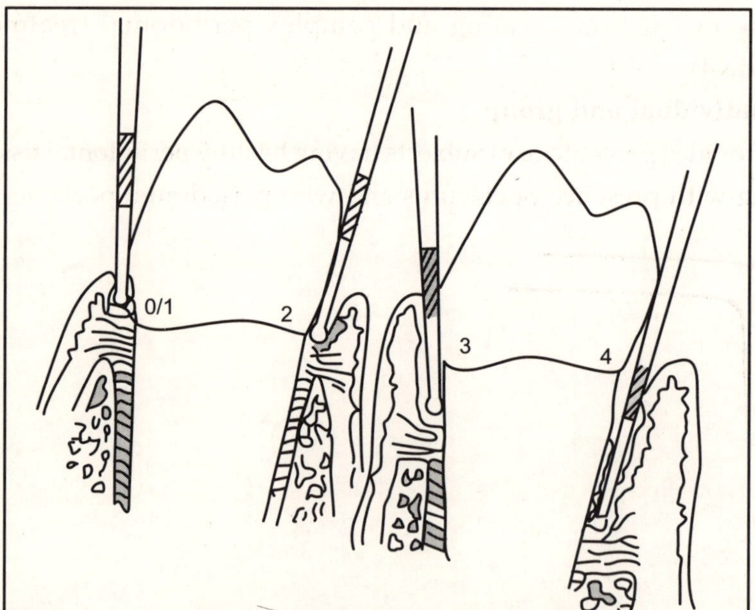

Figure 9.3: Community periodontal index of treatment needs (CPITN). Code – 0 no periodontal diseases (healthy periodontium). Code – 1 bleeding on gentle probing. Code – 2 calculus felt during probing. Code – 3 periodontal pocket depth between 3.5 and 5.5 mm where the black band is visible. Code – 4 periodontal pocket depth where the black band is not visible

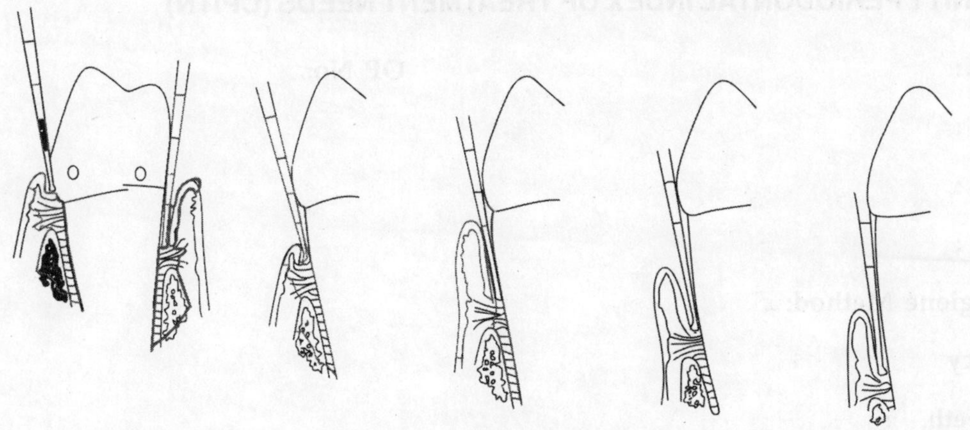

Figure 9.4: Examples of coding for loss of attachment with a CPI probe

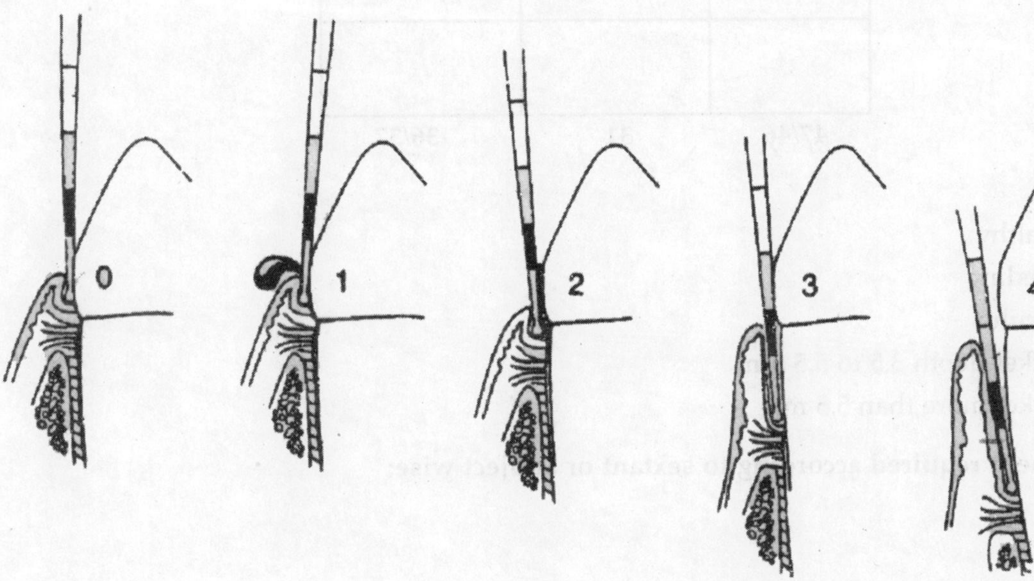

Figure 9.5: Examples of coding according to the community periodontal index, showing the position of the CPI probe

COMMUNITY PERIODONTAL INDEX OF TREATMENT NEEDS (CPITN)

Case No.: **OP No:**

Name :

Age :

Gender :

Oral Hygiene Method:

Frequency :

Index Teeth :

17/16	11	26/27
47/46	31	36/37

Code:

0 – Healthy
1 – Bleeding
2 – Calculus
3 – Pocket depth 3.5 to 5.5 mm
4 – Pocket more than 5.5 mm

Treatment required according to sextant or subject wise:

Staff Signature
Date:

CHAPTER TEN

Dental Fluorosis

DEFINITION (WHO)

Endemic dental fluorosis is a specific disturbance of tooth formation caused by excessive intake of fluoride during the formative period of dentition. Clinical dental fluorosis is characterized by lustreless, Opaque white patches in the enamel, which may become striated, mottled and or pitted or may be stained yellow to dark brown the affected teeth may show a pronounced accentuation of the perikymata and in more severe cases, discrete pits and larger areas of hypoplasia (confluent pitting. of the enamel appear to such an extent that the morphology of the tooth is lost.

CLASSIFICATION OF DENTAL FLUOROSIS

In order to compare the severity and distribution on dental fluorosis in various communities, Dean developed an epidemiological index according to which each tooth is allotted a score and each score is given a corresponding weightage:

Score	Weight
0—Normal	0
1—Questionable	0.5
2—Very mild	1.0
3—Mild	2.0
4—Moderate	3.0
5—Severe	4.0

For each score a corresponding description of the clinical appearance of the tooth was given

Normal: The enamel presents the usual translucent, semivitriform type of structure the surface is smooth, glossy and usually of a pale creamy white colour.

Questionable: The enamel discloses slight aberrations from the translucency of normal enamel, ranging from a few white flecks to occasional white spots this classification is used in those instances where a definite diagnosis of the mildest form of fluorosis not warranted and a classification of "normal" not justified.

Very mild: Small, opaque paper white areas scattered irregularly over the tooth, but involving less than approximately 25 per cent of the tooth surface, frequently included in this classification are teeth showing not more than about 1-2 mm of white opacity at the tip of the summit of the cusps of the bicuspids or second molars.

Mild: The white opaque areas in the enamel surfaces of teeth are more extensive but do not involve as much as 50 per cent of the tooth

Moderate: All enamel surfaces of teeth show marked wear Brown stain is frequently a disfiguring feature.

Severe: Includes teeth formerly classified as "moderately severe" and "severe". All enamel surfaces are affected and hypoplasia is so marked that the general form of the tooth may be altered. The major diagnostic sign of this classification is the discrete or confluent pitting. Brown stains are wide spread and teeth often present a corroded like appearance.

The score assigned to an individual is the one that correspond to the two most severely affected teeth in the individual mouth.

COMMUNITY INDEX OF DENTAL FLUOROSIS (FCI)

On the basis of the number and distribution of the individual scores a community index of dental fluorosis (FCI) could be

$$\text{FCI} = \frac{\text{number of individuals x statistical weight}}{\text{total number of individuals examined}}$$

Example:

Number of persons	*Score*	*Sum of statistical weights*
50	0	0
25	0.5	12.5
15	1	15
10	2	20
5	3	15
5	4	20
Total 110	82.5	82.5

$$\text{FCI} = \frac{82.5}{110} = 0.75$$

Dean stated that: "For public health administrative guidance a community index of dental fluorosis of 0.4 or less is of no concern from the standpoint of mottled enamel per se. when, however, the index rises above health problem warranting increasing consideration."

CHAPTER ELEVEN
Topical Fluorides

AN INDIVIDUALIZED FLUORIDE THERAPY FOR DENTAL CARIES PREVENTION

Fluorides have been proved to be the single most effective weapon in our still limited arsenel of anticaries agents.

Dental profession has also been cognizant of the limitations of fluoridation of community water supply as more than 40 percent of the population of even the best developed countries like USA would be deprived of water fluoridation due to lack of central water supply system.

In India at best 30 percent of population is supplied by central water supply, hence more than 70 percent of population cannot be covered by water fluoridation.

Fortunately for caries suffering humanity various efficient methods of fluoride therapy at the individual level surfaced. In 1941, began an era of topical fluorides when 0.1% NaF was introduced by Bibby, subsequently over the years other fluorides evolved such as SnFg, APF, NaMFP, amine fluorides and varnish containing fluoride.

TWO PERCENT SODIUM FLUORIDE (KNUTSON'S TECHNIQUE)

Milestone studies were conducted by Bibby and Knutson which varied not only in concentration of NaF used but also in the number of applications per year.

After carrying out various studies KNUTSONS FELDMAN recommended a technique for application of NaF. Knutson used 2% sodium fluoride and the technique recommended 4 applications of NaF at weekly intervals in a year and also recommended 3, 7, 11 and 13 years as specific age groups for NaF application.

One disadvantage of the use of Knutson technique is that patient must make 4 visit to the dentist within a relatively short time.

METHOD OF PREPARING 2% SODIUM FLUORIDE

Two percent NaF solution can be prepared by dissolving 20 gms of NaF powder in 1 litre of distilled water in a plastic bottle.

Note: It is essential to store fluoride in plastic bottles because if stored in glass containers, the fluoride ion of solution can react with silica of glass forming SiFg, thus reducing the availability of free active fluorides for anticaries action.

METHOD OF APPLICATION OF 2% NaF ACCORDING TO KNUTSON'S TECHNIQUE

— Initially cleaning and polishing of the teeth is done in only the first of the four applications.

— Upper and lower quadrant are isolated with cotton rolls and the teeth are dried thoroughly.

— 2% NaF is then applied with cotton applicators and is permitted to dry on the teeth for 4 minutes.

The procedure is repeated for the remaining quadrants in the same manner.

After completion of treatment the patient is instructed to avoid eating, drinking or rinsing for 30 minutes, so as to prolong the availability of fluoride ion to react with the tooth surfaces.

Second, third and fourth applications are given at weekly intervals. A full series of four treatments is recommended at age 3, 7,11 and 13.

MECHANISM OF ACTION OF 2% NaF

When NaF is applied topically, it reacts with hydroxy appetite crystals to form CaF_2 which is the dominant product of reaction.

$$Ca_{10}(PO_4)_6(OH)_2 + 20F = 10CaF_2 + 6PO_4^- + 2OH$$

This is due to high concentration of Fluoride in 2% NaF due to which the solubility product of CaF_2 get exceeded fast and this initial rapid reaction is followed by drastic reduction in its rate and the phenomenon is called "choking off". This occurs because once a thick layer of CaF_2 is formed it interferes with the further diffusion of fluoride from the topical fluoride solution to react with hydroxyapatite, Further CaF_2 reacts with hydroxyapatite to form fluoridated hydroxyapatite.

$$CaF_2 + 2Ca_5(PO_4)_3OH = 2Ca_5(PO_4)_3F + Ca(OH)_2$$

This increases the concentration of surface fluoride, thus making the tooth structure more stable, less susceptible to dissolution by adds, interferes with plaque metabolism through anti enzymatic action and also helps in remineralisation of the initial decalcified areas thus showing its manifold anticaries effects.

CARIOSTATIC TOPICAL STANNOUS FLUORIDE: (MUHLER'S TECHNIQUE)

Eight percent STANNOUS FLUORIDE in early 1950's occupied a central role in the saga of preventive dentistry.

Muhler et al in 1947 observed that enamel powders treated with stannous fluoride solution greatly reduced the rate of acid dissolution and in another *in vitro* study found that SnF_2 to be three times more effective than NaF.

METHOD OF PREPARATION OF 8% STANNOUS FLUORIDE

Stannous fluoride solution has to be freshly prepared before use each time as it has no shelf life.

For convenient preparation '0' No. gelatine capsules are priorily filled with 0.8 gm. Powdered SnF_2 and are stored in air tight plastic containers just before application, the content of one capsule is dissolved in 10 ml of distilled water in a plastic container and the solution thus prepared is shaken briskly. The solution is then applied immediately to the teeth. The 10 ml of solution should be sufficient to treat the whole mouth of a single patient. If any remains it should be discarded and not to be used again.

METHOD OF APPLICATION OF 8% SnF_2

— The recommended procedure for topical application of 8% SnF_2 begins with through prophylaxis.
— The teeth are then isolated with cotton rolls and dried preferably with compressed air.
— Either a quadrant or half of the mouth can be treated at one time.
— A freshly prepared 8% solution of SnF_2 is applied continuously to the teeth with cotton applicators so that the teeth are kept moist with the solution for four minutes and a reapplication of the solution to a particular tooth is done every 15 to 30 seconds.
— The recommended frequency of 8% SnF_2 applications is once per year.

MECHANISM OF ACTION OF 8% SNF_2

Muhler reported that when SnF_2 react with hydroxyapatite in addition to fluoride the tin of SnF_2 also reacts with enamel and a new crystalline product gets formed which is different from fluorapitite and this new compound which is stannous trifluorophosphate ($Sn_3F_3PO_4$) is more resistant to decay than enamel.

Note: It is due to this reason that always a freshly prepared SnF_2 solution should be used and the capsule of SnF_2 should be kept in air tight containers. Otherwise the stannous form of Tin gets oxidised to stannic form, thus making the SnF_2 inactive for anticaries action.

Infrared absorption and X-ray diffraction analysis of the reaction of SnF_2 with HA shows that mainly four end products get formed.

Tin hydroxyphosphate ($Sn_2(OH)PO_4$) is formed when SnF_2 is applied in low concentration. Second and main end product which gets formed is Tin-Trifluorophosphate (SnF_3PO_4). At very high concentrations of SnF_2 calcium Trifluorostanate ($Co(SnF_3)_2$) gets formed along with $Sn_3F_4PO_4$ (TTFP).

CaF_2 in low quantity is also the end product both in low and high concentration.

The chemical reaction involved at low level concentration is:

$$Ca_5(PO_4)_3OH + 2SnF_2 \rightarrow 2CaF_2 + Sn_2(OH)PO_4 + Ca_3(POH_2)$$

The chemical reaction involved at high concentration is:

$$Ca_5(PO_4)_3OH + 16\,SnF_2 \rightarrow CaF_2 + 2Sn_3F_3PO_4 + Sn_2(OH)PO_4 + 4CaF_2(SnF_3)$$

CRITICAL APPRAISAL OF ACIDULATED PHOSPHATE FLUORIDE AS A CARIOSTATIC AGENT (BRUDEVOLD'S TECHNIQUE)

The idea of acidulated phosphate fluoride as a topical agent in the prevention of Dental caries emerged with the *in vitro,* investigation of Bibby who reported that as the pH of the NaF solution was lowered, fluoride was absorbed into enamel more effectively.

This statement of Bibby had its inherent limitations as indiscriminate lowering of pH of NaF solution will cause decalcification and demineralization of the enamel thus obviating the fluoride effect.

Brudevold and his co-workers did systematic investigations to find out an optimal fluoride concentration which would provide maximal fluoride deposition while causing minimal decalcification.

One of the practical difficulties of doing the topical application with APF solution is that the teeth must be kept wet with solution for 4 minutes and moreover, APF solution is acidic and sour and bitter in taste so repeated applications necessitates the use of suction thereby minimising its use in the field. This also made multiple chair program by one dentist or auxiliary difficult thereby increasing the chairside time and making this F–application programme more expensive.

To overcome these problems APF gels were introduced. Since with gel fluoride comes in constant contact with teeth, re-application is not required and as it is possible to do self application and with that the cost of application also gets reduced.

Comparing the two i.e., APF solution and APF gel. APF gel though relatively costly readily available as yet have to be imported in India for use but has the advantage of being used as self application.

The APF solution is cheap can be prepared easily but has to be applied topically by a dentist or the auxiliary staff.

METHOD OF PREPARATION OF APF SOLUTION/GEL

Acidulated phosphate fluoride usually contains 1.23 percent fluoride in 0.1 M phosphoric acid at a pH of 3.0 and is stable with long shelf life when stored in opaque plastic bottles.

It is prepared by dissolving 20 gm of NaF in I litre of 0.1 M phosphoric add and to this is added 50 percent hydrofluoric acid to adjust the pH at 2.0 and F concentration at 1.23 percent.

For the preparation of APF gel, a gelling agent Methyle cellulose or hydroxyethyl cellulose is to be added to the solution and the pH is to be adjusted between.

METHOD OF APPLICATION OF APF

After thorough prophylaxes, the teeth are isolated with cotton rolls on both lingual and buccal sides dried and APF solution is continuously and repeatedly applied with cotton applicators and the teeth are kept moist for four minutes. Floss may be drawn through each inter - proximal embrassures to ensure wetting of these surfaces. The recommended frequency of APF topical application is semiannually.

APF gel may be applied in the same manner as topical solution but APF gel can be used by self application procedure and children can be trained for this. A variety of self reusable or disposable trays in various sizes together with sponge like tray - liners are available.

MECHANISM OF ACTION

Aasenden and Brudevold and Mccann reported that the tooth enamel acquired larger amounts of fluoride with deeper penetration when pretreated with 'dilute phosphoric add before being exposed to F solution.

The author further reported that when APF is applied on the teeth. It initially leads to dehydration and shrinkage in the volume of HAP crystals which further on hydrolysis forms an intermediate product called dicalcium phosphate dehydrate (DCPD).

This DCPD which is highly reactive with 'F' penetrate into title crystals more deeply through the openings produced by shrinkage and leads to formation of FA.

$Ca_5(PO_4)_3\,OH + 4H^+ \leftrightarrows 5Ca^{++} + 3HPO_4^- + H_2O^-$

$Ca^{++} + HPO_4^- \leftrightarrows^{OH^-} Ca\,HPO_4\,2H_2O$ (Dicalcium Phospate Dihydration)

$5CaHPO_4\,2H_2O \leftrightarrows^{F^-} Ca_5(P04)_3F + 2HPO_4^-$

The amount and depth of F' deposited as FAP would be dependent on the amount and depth at which DCPD gets formed. Since for the conversion of whole of DCPD so formed into FAP, deeper penetration and continuous supply of F is required. So APF has to be applied every 30 seconds and the teeth be kept wet for 4 minutes.

TOPICAL FLUORIDES APPLICATION – EXERCISES

Sl. No.	*Name of the Patient*	*Age*	*Sex*	*Name of the F. used*	*Time applied*	*Signature of staff*

CHAPTER TWELVE

Pit and Fissure Sealants

DEFINITION

A pit and fissure resin sealant is an organic polymer that bonds to the enamel surface mainly by mechanical retention. It acts as a physical barrier to prevent oral bacteria and their nutrients from collecting within pit or fissure and creating the acid environment essential to the initiation of dental caries.

CRITERIA FOR SELECTING TEETH FOR SEALANT PLACEMENT

Several Factors are Considered

A. *Location of Pits and Fissures:* Sealants are indicated for permanent and primary teeth that have pits and fissures. These include occlusal pits and fissures, facial pits, palatal pits.

B. *Contour of pits and Fissures:* Sealants are indicated especially for teeth with deep, narrow pits and fissures. Teeth with shallow and well coalesced pits and fissures are less likely to become carious - because/they are more accessible for plaque control.

C. *Relation to Eruption:* Applications should be made as soon as possible following eruption when applications are delayed, caries may start, the surface no longer considered for sealant.

D. *Relation to Dental Caries: When* there are current carious lesions and previous restoration, newly erupted teeth should be treated promptly. Incipient pit and fissure caries is arrested by sealant placement.

E. *Age:* Age of patient may have particular significance. Application of a sealant to caries free occlusal surface during early teenage years, when caries rates are high, may prove beneficial to the individual (3-4 years - sealing eligible decidous teeth).

F. *Prevention Program:* Sealant application should be part of complete prevention program, not an isolated procedure.

CONTRAINDICATION

- Patient behaviour does not permit use of adequate dry field techniques throughout the procedure.
- There is an open occlusal carious lesion.
- Caries exist on other surfaces of the same tooth.

BACKGROUND ON SEALANT

Three different kinds of plastics have been used as occlusal sealants.

1. Polyurethanes
2. Cyanoacrylates
3. Bisphenol A-glycidylmethylacrylate(BIS-GMA)

Polvurethanes

Were first to appear.

They proved to be too soft and totally disintegrated in the mouth after 2 to 3 months. During the time that plastics adhered to the tooth fluoride continually leached to increase the concentration of fluoride in the enamel.

Cyanoacrylates

Have also tried as sealants, but they too disintegrated after slightly longer period of time. The (ADA) council of dental materials did not recomend the cynoacrylates for routine use in dentistry because formaldehyde was formed as part of biodegradation in oral fluids.

BIS-GMA

(Bisphenol A—glycidyl methyl acrylate) is now the sealant of choice. It is the mixture of BIS-GMA and methyl methacrylate. Its successful use was first reported by Buonocore.

The Commercial Products Accepted by ADA

- Concise brand white sealant
- Deltan clear and tinted
- Helioseal white
- Nerva seal
- Visio seal

Polymerizing of the Sealant

The liquid plastic is called monomer. When monomer is acted upon by the catalyst repeating chemical bonds begin to form increasing the number and complexity as the hardening process proceeds. Finally, the resultant hard product is known as polymer.

Two methods have been employed to catalyse polymerisation.

1. Light curing by a photopolymerisation: Use of either an UV or visible blue light.
2. Self curing or chemical or autopolymerisation: Where monomer and catalyst are mixed together.

Requisites for Sealant Retention

For sealant retention it is necessary that surface of tooth.

- have maximum surface area
- have deep irregular pits and fissures
- be clean
- be absolutely dry at time of sealant placement and uncontaminated with saliva residue.

Increasing the Surface Area

Sealant do not bond directly to the teeth. Instead, they are retained mainly by adhesive forces. To increase the surface area which in turn increases the adhesive potential, tooth conditioners called (etchants) that are composed of 30 to 50 percent. Concentration of phosphoric acid are placed prior to placement of sealant. The etchant may be liquid or gel form. If there are any etched areas on the tooth surface not covered by sealant or if not retained—normal appearance returns to tooth within one hour.

Pits and Fissure Depth

Deep, irregular pits and fissures offer a much more favourable surface contour for sealant retention compared to broad, shallow fossae. The deeper fissure protect the plastic sealant from shear forces occurring as result of masticatory movements.

Surface Cleanliness

All heavy stain, deposits and debris should be off the occlusal surface before applying the sealant. Methods of cleaning—prophylaxis, some advocate use of pumice and water slurry. The use of an air polish is another cleaning operation. H_2O_2 (hydrogen peroxide) has also been tried as a cleaning agent but has the disadvantage that it produce a precipitate on the enamel surface.

Dryness

The teeth must dry at the time of sealant placement, since the present Sealants are hydroplastic. The pressure of saliva on the tooth is even more detrimental than water, since its organic components interpose a barrier between the tooth and the sealant of moisture is present that will prevent adhesion of the sealant to enamel.

Dry field can be maintained by use of rubber dam, employment of cotton rolls, placement of bibulous pads over the opening of parotid duct and use of other armamentarium.

Application of Sealant

Each quadrant should be treated separately. General directions are described here in sequence. The success of treatment depends on precision in the techniques of application.

Cleaning the Tooth Surface

For successful sealant retention in pits is fissures add etch technique is used.

Purposes

- Remove deposits and debris
- Permit maximum contact of the sealant with enamel surface.

Patient with no Stain or Calculus

a. Suction the pits and fissuers with high volume evacuator
b. Use a sharp explore to dig out debris and bacteria
c. Suction again to remove loosened material
d. Additional cleaning is not necessary.

Cleaning Effect of Acid Etch Conditioner

The acid etch conditioner removes a shallow layer of enamel. At the same time, plaque, surface pellicle and sub-surface pellicle are removed. Additional cleaning procedures are not necessary.

Cleansing Agent

When-indicated because of heavy dental stains, fine pumice and water are used with a pointed polishing brush in a slow-speed hand piece.

1. Use only the pumice and water mix. Oil and fluoride must not be present. Commercial polishing pastes are contraindicated because frequently they contain glycerin, oils, flavouring agents, and fluorides that can interfere with bonding.
2. Apply the pumice mixture with a rotating pointed bristle brush. 'Jab' the bristles into the pits and fissures to remove as much stain and debris as possible. Rinse and suction clean with an explorer tip.

Isolate the Tooth

a. Purposes of isolation
   1. Keep the tooth clean and dry for optimal action and bonding of sealant.
   2. To eliminate contamination by saliva and moisture from breath.

b. Rubber dam
   1. Rubber dam application is the method of choice because the most complete isolation is obtained.
   2. It is essential when profuse saliva and overactive tongue and oral muscles make retraction and consistent maintenance of dry, clean field.

Dry the Tooth

a. Purpose
   1. Prepare the tooth for the conditioning
   2. Prevent dilution and contamination of the conditioner.

b. Use only dry, oil free, clean air
   Air dry atleast for 10 seconds

Apply Conditioner for Enamel Etching

a. Purpose
   1. Creates surface irregularities to increase the area of retention.
   2. To make the enamel rods accessible to the adhesive.
   3. Remove bacterial plaque and pellicle.

b. Conditioner
   1. Apply phosphoric acid (37 to 50%) with a brush, cotton pellet or plastic sponge.
   2. Note the time or start timer. Total application time is as follows:
      a. I minute: permanent teeth
      b. 2 minutes: primary teeth
      c. 4 minutes: fluorosed teeth
   3. Place gel over the surface and leave undisturbed.
   4. Do gentle dabbing

Rinse Thoroughly

a. Purpose
   1. To remove excess acid
   2. To prevent saliva from reaching the etched surface
b. Procedure
   1. Do not permit the patient to rinse or expectorate.
   2. Clear the water in the tubing of air/water syringe by releasing water into a sink.
   3. Hold wide aspirator tip between tooth and cotton.
   4. Rinse thoroughly (10 to 15 seconds) for solution; 30 seconds for gel.
   5. Evacuate excess water from entire area immediately after rinsing.
   6. Maintain dry area.
   7. If accidental contamination with saliva occur, wash, dry and etch again for 10 seconds, wash and dry to prepare for next step.
c. Examine the surface:
   The etched surface should be a dull, chalky, white when it is not, repeat the application of conditioner step-by-step.

Dry the Tooth Thoroughly Again

Procedure

1. Dry the tooth thoroughly for 15 to 30 seconds per tooth, use only clean, dry oil free air.
2. Do not blow saliva onto the etched surface.

Apply the Sealant

a. Follow manufactures instruction

b. Placement:
   i. Do the posterior most tooth First
   ii. Do only two teeth per mix
c. Application
   i. Use disposable applicator
   ii. Flow the sealant first to pit and fissure that has maximum depth, avoid marginal ridge and cusp tip.

Fluoride and Sealant

I. Topical application in conjunction with sealant when used, fluoride must be applied before the conditioner or after the sealant. It should not be applied between there two steps because the bond strength may be reduced between the sealant and etched enamel surface.

II. Combined preventive program:

Sealant are part of a total preventive program. Although sealant is applicable for occlusal surfaces fluoride application and other fluoride resources for self-administration are necessary for all other surfaces.

PIT AND FISSURE SEALANTS

Sl. No.	*Name of the patient*	*Age*	*Sex*	*Sealant used*	*Signature of staff*

CHAPTER THIRTEEN

Plaque Control Programmes

Plaque is a tenacious adherent material deposited on to the tooth surface and on the soft tissue or oral cavity. Its main composition is made of bacteria, organic and inorganic materials.

The patients (adult/child) having bad oral hygiene are selected for this study. They are advised to attend the clinic with their tooth brush, tooth paste and other inter dental cleansing agents. (Dental floss, tooth pick, proxa-brush, etc.).

Any one of the below mentioned enclosing agents are used for exhibiting plaque: Solution. Basic Euschin, Potassium Iodide, Merchurochrome, Alpha-Plac, Dis-Plac, etc. Wafers: Erythrocin (FDC Red 3) 3-15 mg tables, etc.

METHOD

1. The individual is asked to chew the disclosing tablet for a minute and swish with water (or any other solution to be applied).
2. The disclosed plaque is shown to the patient in the mirror situated near a wash basin. The harmful effects of plaque is explained to the individual.
3. The patient is shown proper method of using brush and other inter dental cleansing agents to remove the plaque.
4. The individual is allowed to remove plaque with all the above aids.
5. After rinsing, again the remaining plaque is disclosed 1 to show areas to be concentrated upon.
6. Proper guidance and instructions are given.
7. The exercise can be repeated at weekly intervals till the individual develops the skill of proper brushing.

PLAQUE CONTROL PROGRAMME

Sl. No.	*Name of the patient*	*Age*	*Sex*	*Disclosing solution used*	*Signature of staff*

CHAPTER FOURTEEN

Dental Health Education Materials

Prepare Dental Health Education Materials like charts, models, booklets, palmlets, cartoons, stories, street plays, skits, imprinted formates or CD, OHP sheets, models, i.e. three-dimensional format which gives details about.

1. Functions of teeth and its associated parts.
2. Structure of teeth and its associated parts.
3. Common dental and oral diseases.
4. Treatment procedures of dental and oral diseases.
5. Prevention of dental and oral diseases.
6. Promotion of dental and oral health.

CHAPTER FIFTEEN

Field Programme Reports

DENTAL CAMPS

Dental camps play an important role in extending dental health to rural people, school children and other needy groups.

In some camps, all individuals can utilise the dental treatment where the facilities are provided by the organisers of the camp. In others the dental camps are organised only for specific selected groups, e.g. school, institutions, etc.

Certain camps are only preventive in nature (e.g. Dental Health Education) and some others are screening for oral problems and in few treatment is also provided.

Mostly these camps are organised with the help of concerned authorities or with the help of voluntary organisations.

The students should attend dental camps arranged by the department.

He/She should be able to:

1. Understand the great need of providing dental treatment to the poor and needy.
2. Organise the camp in association with voluntary organisations or any other relevant authorities.
3. Improve and learn public relations, planning, public health administration and man power utilisation.
4. Organise and deliver the basic dental treatment both preventive and curative with minimum available facilities in camp area.
5. Appreciate the need or imparting dental knowledge of the public in dental camps.
6. Understand the purpose of serving the handicapped groups such as blind, deaf, dumb, etc.

DENTAL HEALTH EDUCATION

The importance of health education in dental profession need not be stressed. Most of the oral and dental diseases are preventable by individual actions. The lack of knowledge added with ignorance forms the basis for the increasing trends of oral diseases.

The primary objective of health education is to persuade the people.

1. To adopt and sustain healthy life practices.
2. To use judiciously and wisely health services available to them.
3. To take their own decisions both individually and collectively to improve their health status and environment.

DEFINITION

"Dental health education is a process that informs motivates and helps people to adopt and maintain health life practices and lifestyles, advocates environmental changes as needed to achieve maximum status of Oral health.

The candidate should be able to appreciate the need of "Health Education and should learn to deliver the educational lectures under the guidance of teaching staff.

THE STUDENT MUST DEVELOP

a. Confidence to deliver speech both in English and their own regional language.
b. Efficiency of using appropriate impressive language and subject matter to different strata of groups, e.g. children, officials, villagers, nurses, etc.
c. Skill of educating with or without the help of audiovisual aids and motivating the people.
d. The knowledge of conducting Dental Health Exhibitions.

FIELD PROGRAMMES

(A) DENTAL CAMPS

Sl. No.	*Date*	*Place of Camp*	*TREATMENT RENDERED (No.)*			*Dental Health Education*	*Staff Signature*
			Oral Prophylaxis	*Restorations Perm.*	*Extractions*		

(A) DENTAL CAMPS
(REPORT)

FIELD PROGRAMMES

(B) A VISIT TO WATER PURIFICATION PLANT

Place of visit

Date of visit

DETAILED REPORT OF THE VISIT

FIELD PROGRAMMES

(C) A VISIT TO PRIMARY HEALTH CENTRE/SCHOOLS

Place of visit

Date of visit

DETAILED REPORT OF THE VISIT

FIELD PROGRAMMES

(D) A VISIT TO SLUM AREA/INSTITUTIONS/HOLISTIC HEALTH CENTRES

Place of visit

Date of visit

DETAILED REPORT OF THE VISIT

FIELD PROGRAMMES

(E) A VISIT TO DENTAL CLINICS

DETAILED REPORT OF THE VISIT

Index